Australian Tea Tree Oil
FIRST AID
HANDBOOK

101 Plus Ways to Use Tea Tree Oil

2nd Edition

Cynthia Olsen

LOTUS
PRESS

Twin Lakes, Wisconsin

COPYRIGHT 1999 KALI PRESS

Cover & page design: Paul Bond, Art & Soul Design

Editing & page composition: Patrick Seger and Cary Diane Ellis

Illustration: Christopher S. Gerlach

Olsen, Cynthia B.
      Australian tea tree oil handbook : 101 plus ways to use tea tree oil / Cynthia Olsen. — 2nd ed.
      p. cm.
      Includes index.

      1. Melaleuca alternifolia oil--Therapeutic use.
I. Title.

    RM666.M357047   615'.32376
                    QBI99-658
ISBN 10: 1-8909-4102-6   ISBN 13: 978-1-8909-4102-4

First published in 1991 by Kali Press

Second US Edition published by:
Lotus Press, PO Box 325, Twin Lakes, WI 53181
Email: lotuspress@lotuspress.com
Website: www.lotuspress.com

Printed in the United States of America

Contents

DEDICATION   vi

INTRODUCTION   1

HEAD   5

Cleansing Hair and Follicles   5

Dandruff   6

Dry or Oily Hair & Itchy Scalp   6

Earaches   6

Ear Infections   6

Head Cold   7

Head Lice (pediculus humans capitis)   7

Nasal Ulcers   8

Sinusitis   8

FACE   9

Acne   9

After Shave and Waxing   10

Canker Sores   10

Chapped Lips   10

Cold Sores (Herpes Simplex I)   11

Styes   11

TEETH   13

Gingivitis   14

Mouthwash Formula   15

Sore Gums, Bad Breath and Plaque   15

Toothache   16

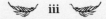

Toothbrush Care   16

THROAT & CHEST   17

Bronchial Congestion/Bronchitis   17
Emphysema   17
Sore Throat   18
Coughs   18
Thrush   19
Laryngitis   19

BODY   21

Arthritis   21
Bruises   22
Burns (minor)   22
Dermatitis   23
Eczema   24
Hives   24
Minor Cuts and Abrasions   24
Muscle Aches   24
Psoriasis   25
Ringworm, Scalp   25
Ringworm, Skin   26
Warts   26

LEGS & FEET   27

Athletes Foot (Tinea)   27
Blisters   27
Corns and Calluses   28
Diabetic Gangrene   28
Gout   29
Leg Ulcers   29

Plantars Warts   30

PERSONAL HYGIENE   31
Bladder Infection (Cystitis)   31
Hemorrhoids   32
Herpes Lesions (simplex type II)   33
Jock Itch   33
Ovarian Cysts   33
Vaginitis   34
Waxing Bikini Area/Legs   35

BEAUTY CARE   37
Acne Mask   37
Body Lotion   38
Body Smoother   38
Dry Brushing   38
Dry Skin   39
Facial Mask - Oily Skin   39
Nail Soak   40
Nail Stains   40
Nail Infections (Perionychia)   40

HOME CARE & ON THE ROAD   41
SECTION I: HOUSEHOLD CLEANING   42
Author's notes   42
Disinfectant/ Cleanser   42
Essential Oil   42
Food Grade Hydrogen Peroxide   42
Alice's Wonder Spray   43
Chemicals in Cleaning Products   44
Dishwashers   45

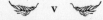

Household Cleaning Solution   45
Plants   45
Washing Machines   46

SECTION II: HOME NURSING CARE   46

Bedsores   46
Hand Disinfectant   46
Humidifier   47
Mood/Memory Pick Me Upper   47
Room Freshener   47
Vaporizer   47

AROMATHERAPY   49
Bath Salts   50
Deep Hair Conditioner   50
Deodorizer   50
Dry Skin   50
Hair Rinse - For Scalp   51
Massage   51
Perfume Body Mist   51
Vaporizer   51

BABY & CHILD CARE   53
Chicken Pox   53
Colds   54
Cradle Cap - Dermatitis   54
Diaper Cleanser   54
Diaper Rash (Nappy Rash)   54
Earaches/Ear Infections   55
Heat and Skin Rash   55
Impetigo   55

Insect Bites   55

Measles   56

Room Deodorizer and Disinfectant   57

Sore Breasts (From Breast Feeding)   57

Tonsillitis   57

OUTDOORS/CAMPING   59

Blisters   59

Fire Ant Bites   59

Insect Bites and Stings   60

Insect Repellent   60

Leeches   60

Poison Ivy/Poison Oak/Poison Sumac   61

Sandfleas   61

Splinters   61

Sprains   61

Sunburn   62

Ticks   62

Letter from a camper   63

APPENDIX   65

Salve Recipes   65

Water Miscible Mixtures   67

Storage   68

Precautions   68

Material Safety Data Sheet   69

Tea Tree Information   71

INDEX   75

ABOUT THE AUTHOR   83

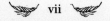

Dedication

I dedicate this book to my beloved sister Patricia,
who I honor for her courage, beauty, strength and faith.

In childhood you held me by my hand as I hold you
in my heart today and always.

Introduction

As we step into the next millennium, remember to bring along your Tea Tree Oil (*Melaleuca alternifolia*). Tea Tree Oil has become increasingly more known and used as a first aid remedy for a number of skin ailments. The scientific research, in Australia and in the U.S. have confirmed the efficacy in treating bacterial and fungal skin infections. To quote Dr Paul Belaiche, Chief of Phytotherapy Department at the University of Paris, France, "The Essential oil of *Melaleuca* has entered the team of major essential oils and emerges as an antiseptic and antifungal weapon of the first order in phyto-aromatherapy."

Natural medicine is becoming more mainstream. The baby boomers now make up a large portion of consumers in the natural products industry. Sales of herbs in natural food stores and chain stores rose over 20% between 1994 and 1996, and are continuing that trend. There is more scientific and medical research that confirms the efficacy of herbs. Prevention Magazine and NBC News in recent polls indicate that one-third of Americans purchase herbal products.

The Australian Bundjalung Aborigines intuitively knew how to use the oil by grinding the leaves into a paste and applying it on bites, cuts and burns. Their folk wisdom has been passed down for generations, and has been validated through scientific research.

More recently, Tea Tree Oil is being recognized worldwide for commercial uses in many products including suppositories, household cleaning, baby care, massage formulas, foot balm, deodor-

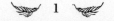

ant, bath oil, sunscreen, insect repellent, toothpaste, mouthwash, soap and veterinarian products.

In looking for Tea Tree Oil products one can visit their local heath food store, body care and herbal shops. Tea Tree is now making appearances in mainstream stores, drugstores, supermarkets and mass-market retailers. Be sure you are purchasing one hundred percent *Melaleuca alternifolia*.

Personally, I have used Tea Tree Oil for many years and will continue to do so. I have introduced this marvelous essential oil to my family and friends. When I travel, Tea Tree Oil comes along. I realized I could do with one bottle of Tea Tree Oil what three-quarters of the items in the drugstore do.

The second edition of the Handbook is packed full of first aid applications for children, adults, home care providers, campers, and the elderly. The uses are still from head to toe and have been expanded upon. I always welcome and encourage suggestions and more ideas from my readers.

Tea Tree Oil is still one of the finest gifts from nature and has earned its praiseworthy reputation as the" Medicine Kit in a bottle."

Cynthia B. Olsen
Colorado, 1999

ff We are a German family including one dog and we got introduced to Tea Tree Oil 3 years ago. This wonderful oil is an extraordinary medicine. We are very grateful for all the recipes named in your book. We use it frequently for all kinds of illnesses; colds, sore throats, inhalation and ear infections (my father suffered from terrible painful ear infections); since we use Tea Tree Oil according to these recipes, they vanished completely.

In addition to these treatments we apply it for muscle massages, baths and for disinfecting in general. It is also good and effective against warts. This oil helps us a great deal and we will always keep it in our home pharmacy and travel bag. This oil is an all around medicine that facilitates our life, and is much cheaper than all the chemical stuff.

We often use Tea Tree Oil to kill ticks that attack our little dog from time to time. Fleas also do not appear since we wash him regularly with a Tea Tree Oil shampoo. **"**

Ana Kreisz, Germany

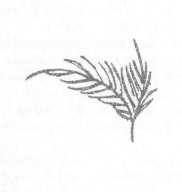

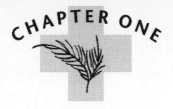

Head

There are commercial Tea Tree Oil shampoos in the market place. You may use those or a natural shampoo that contains no additives or preservatives. Sodium laurel sulphate and propyl alcohol are considered carcinogenic, so check the ingredients carefully and look for healthy alternatives. If you can't pronounce the word, check it out! Tea Tree Oil helps keep the scalp clean, preventing dryness, dandruff and thinning hair.

CLEANSING HAIR AND FOLLICLES

Supplies: Natural shampoo, Tea Tree Oil and vegetable oil.

Remedy: Use a Tea Tree Oil shampoo (usually found in natural food stores or from various Tea Tree manufacturers), or add 10-20 drops of Tea Tree Oil to any shampoo; use daily or alternate with another natural shampoo. Rubbing a few drops of Tea Tree Oil directly into the scalp will help unblock hair follicles.

DANDRUFF

Condition: Dandruff is a common condition in which the scalp becomes dry and itchy and the top layer of skin starts to flake.

Remedy: Follow directions above. Leave shampoo on for a minute or so before rinsing.

DRY OR OILY HAIR & ITCHY SCALP

Remedy: Apply 5 to 10 drops of Tea Tree Oil directly onto hair strands or massage into scalp; also follow *Cleansing Hair Treatment*, page 5.

EARACHES

Condition: Passages leading from the nose to the throat become enlarged, inflamed and painful.

Supplies: Tea Tree Oil, olive oil, dropper and cotton.

Remedy: Warm 1/4 cup of olive oil with 4-5 drops of Tea Tree Oil; drop small amount gently into ear, tilting head to one side for a minute, then repeat other ear if necessary. Put small piece of cotton gently in ear to absorb oil. Repeat remedy until improved.

NOTE: Always dilute Tea Tree Oil before using in ear canal. Be careful not to use any sharp instruments, which could do damage to the ear canal.

EAR INFECTIONS

Condition: My middle daughter had recurring ear infections when she was young. It seems she would get "swimmer's ear" when she was in the water for long periods of time. This remedy may require larger doses of Tea Tree Oil.

Supplies: Tea Tree Oil, olive or almond oil.

Remedy: Start with 1/4 cup olive or almond oil, and add 5 drops of Tea Tree Oil. If the infection persists, increase Tea Tree Oil to 25 drops to a tablespoon of olive or almond oil.

HEAD COLD

Condition: A most uncomfortable feeling, which affects nasal and sinus passages, accompanied by pain and tenderness.

Supplies: Tea Tree Oil, vaporizer and steam inhaler pot.

Remedy: Add 10 drops of Tea Tree Oil to 4 cups of water, drape towel over pot and inhale. At night add 10 drops of Tea Tree Oil to a vaporizer. You can also rub a few drops of Tea Tree Oil on the nose and forehead areas.

HEAD LICE *(PEDICULUS HUMANS CAPITIS)*

Condition: Parents have called and expressed concern regarding outbreaks of lice infestation, which seem to occur after the summer vacation at the beginning of school in the fall. Concerned moms and dads say the school nurse suggests a chemically based treatment. Head lice are highly contagious and can spread very quickly. Lice can be very tenacious and often difficult to eradicate; therefore, combs, brushes, linens and other personal items must be disinfected thoroughly.

Supplies: Tea Tree Oil, shampoo, glycerin, fine tooth comb and 190 proof vodka or everclear (not to be consumed)! Vodka is known for its cleansing properties. I have a friend who uses it as her general cleanser throughout her home and office.

Remedy: Add 10-20 drops of Tea Tree Oil to an ounce of your

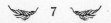

shampoo. Massage into hair, leave on 10 minutes, rinse; repeat procedure once a day until the area is totally clear of eggs and lice. To soak combs, brushes, and linens use a water soluble formula: 1/2 ounce Tea Tree Oil mixed with 1 ounce of glycerin, 2 ounces of vodka and 1 ounce of water. This solution can also be used on the scalp. Add 20 drops of Tea Tree Oil to the washing machine.

NASAL ULCERS

Condition: An open sore or lesion of the mucous membrane accompanied by sloughing of inflamed tissue.

Supplies: Tea Tree Oil and cotton swabs.

Remedy: Dab 2-3 drops of Tea Tree Oil directly onto infected area; apply with cotton swab.

SINUSITIS

Condition: An inflammation of one or more of the mucus-lined air spaces. It is often caused by infection spreading from the nose or allergies. Symptoms may include headache, tenderness and fever. My favorite gadget is the *steam inhaler* which is portable enough to travel with.

Supplies: Tea Tree Oil, bowl, facial steamer, vaporizer, hot cloth.

Remedy: Heat a pot of water on stove. Add 5-10 drops of Tea Tree Oil. Tent your face with a towel, lean over and allow the steam to fill your face and inhale gently. Do not get too close to the steam. You can also sprinkle several drops of the Tea Tree Oil onto a hot, wet cloth and place it over the nose for 5 minutes. At night use the vaporizer by adding 10 drops of Tea Tree Oil to the water. Add 3 drops into the reservoir and inhale for 5 minutes.

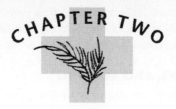

CHAPTER TWO

Face

ACNE

Condition: Acne is just as embarrassing to menopausal adults as it is to teenagers. As the skin is the largest organ, when the body releases toxins and other impurities, the skin erupts. Good nutrition and proper rest, meditation and exercise play a vital role in good skin care.

Supplies: Tea Tree Oil, witch hazel, chamomile and calendula.

Remedy: Use a soapless cleanser, as soap dries and clogs pores; excess scrubbing actually stimulates oil gland production which increases skin blemishes. Avoid any mineral oils such as petroleum jelly as these products will clog the skin. Use a toner that doesn't contain alcohol. Add 5-10 drops of Tea Tree Oil to your toner, or add to 4 ounces of witch hazel and 2-3 drops of calendula or chamomile. Smooth on face. Next, either purchase a Tea Tree Oil acne formula, and add 10 drops of Tea Tree Oil, or apply 3 drops of Tea Tree Oil to infected area twice daily. Add Tea Tree Oil to facewash and add Tea Tree Oil (60 drops) to a natural moisturizing cream (1/4-cup); apply twice daily. Add 15 drops of Tea Tree Oil to 1/2 ounce of a non-drying facewash. (*Beauty without Cruelty Extra Gentle Cleansing Milk™* is one of my favorites).

AFTER SHAVE AND WAXING

Supplies: Tea Tree Oil, aloe vera gel and glycerin.

Remedy: *(after waxing)* I have personally tried this method for extra sensitive areas. It works! I find Aloe Vera gel and glycerin (purchased at drugstore or health store) to be an excellent soothing additive to the Tea Tree Oil.

Remedy: *(after shaving)* Apply a few drops of Tea Tree Oil or Tea Tree cream. Redness usually subsides within a day. Tea Tree Oil can be applied onto razor blade while shaving, to help cut down on nicks. Apply a few drops of pure Tea Tree Oil or Tea Tree cream as an after shave, to act as an antiseptic and eliminate ingrown hairs. Add 5 drops of Tea Tree Oil to 1 tablespoon of aloe vera gel. Smooth over shaved area.

CANKER SORES

Remedy: Gently apply a few drops of Tea Tree Oil directly to infected area with a cotton swab, twice daily. Also add 3 drops to a tumbler of water, swish around mouth. Do not swallow.

My eldest daughter gets these often; especially when she was wearing her braces.

CHAPPED LIPS

Living in a high altitude climate, I always carry lip balm with me, especially while hiking, camping and snow skiing. Adding Tea Tree Oil improves my chapped lip care.

Supplies: Tea Tree Oil moisturizing cream or salve.

Remedy: Apply Tea Tree Oil moisturizing cream or salve.

COLD SORES *(HERPES SIMPLEX 1)*

Condition: A viral infection causing inflammation of the skin, usually on mouth or lips, and characterized by collections of small blisters. Lysine vitamin supplements are recommended if you are prone to reoccurring bouts.

Supplies: Tea Tree Oil and cotton swabs.

Remedy: Gently apply a few drops of Tea Tree Oil directly to infected area with a cotton swab twice daily. To help prevent breakout, apply at onset.

STYE *(HORDEOLUM)*

Condition: An acute localized pyogenic infection of one or more of the glands; generally affecting the eye area. Staphylococci usually are responsible. Recurrence is common.

Supplies: Tea Tree Oil, bowl.

Remedy: Place face over a bowl of hot water to which 5 drops of Tea Tree Oil has been added; steam for 5 minutes.

> *WARNING: It is advisable not to apply oil directly to the eye area; as it will sting and may become irritated. If Tea Tree Oil gets into eyes, wash immediately with cold water.*

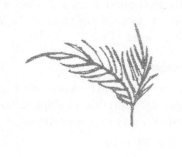

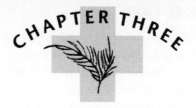

CHAPTER THREE

Teeth

A friend offered this amazing testimonial. "I learned about the amazing healing applications of Tea Tree Oil. One area that particularly interested me was dental application. At the age of 65, I was suffering from receding and bleeding gums. I purchased some Tea Tree Oil and decided to put it to the test. I took the Tea Tree Oil to my dentist and had a full checkup. I told him that I was going to rinse my mouth out twice a day with three drops of Tea Tree Oil in a small cup of water, for about 3-5 minutes. I must tell you that my dentist would get blood at almost every place on my gums. I also gave up flossing. The plan was to have an extensive checkup after 30 days.

My first 30 day checkup showed immediate improvement. My dentist could draw blood in only 6 spots. In 60 days, there was no bleeding at all, even with the gums deeply gouged. After 13 months of treatment, the gums stopped bleeding and the receding gums had returned to normal. The dentist said that the plaque and calculus had been reduced by 75-80%. Tea Tree Oil saved my teeth!"

BASIC DENTAL CARE

Condition: If you clean your teeth properly, and follow nutritional eating habits, you should have healthy gums and strong teeth into your elder years. Sometimes, there aren't enough hours in a day to accomplish all we would like, so we compromise on certain things. Try as I might to brush my teeth for a full 2 minutes twice a day, gargle and floss, it doesn't always get done. Here are some problems that can be greatly reduced using Tea Tree Oil, which fights infectious microorganisms that destroy tissues, cause plaque, receding gums and tarter deposits.

Supplies: Tea Tree Oil and Tea Tree Oil toothpaste, floss, Sonicare, toothbrush and mouthwash

The following herbs may be mixed with Tea Tree Oil:

> Burdock: for its antibiotic properties
>
> Horsetail: contains silicon, provides support to gums
>
> Myrrh: has firming effect on gums
>
> Neem: antimicrobial, helps prevents plaque

There are several natural toothpastes on the market, which contain some of these ingredients; or they may be added.

GINGIVITIS

Condition: Plaque buildup creating inflammation of the gums, redness, swelling, and bleeding.

Supplies: Tea Tree Oil, Tea Tree Oil mouthwash and sea salt.

Remedy: Rub swollen and sore areas of gum with Tea Tree Oil.

Add 3-5 drops of Tea Tree Oil to small glass of water, swish around mouth, twice daily. Apply several drops of Tea Tree Oil directly onto your toothpaste, and brush for at least 2 minutes. Floss, and gargle with a Tea Tree Oil mouthwash. You may also put 5 drops of Tea Tree Oil into a small glass of water, add a pinch of sea salt (contains trace minerals which help remineralize teeth) and gargle.

MOUTHWASH FORMULA

Supplies: Tea Tree Oil and mouthwash.

Remedy: Add 3-5 drops of Tea Tree Oil to 1 ounce of your mouthwash, shake well. Many mouthwashes contain alcohol, which will help to disperse the Tea Tree Oil.

SORE GUMS, BAD BREATH AND PLAQUE

Condition: Plaque is a gummy film that coats the surface of teeth. If not removed every 24 to 36 hours, the bacteria produce toxins that cause inflamed, swollen gums that bleed easily.

Supplies: Tea Tree Oil, baking soda, Tea Tree Oil dental floss and cotton swab.

Remedy: Add 3-5 drops to water and use as a mouthwash twice daily. Brush with Tea Tree Oil toothpaste or add a few drops of Tea Tree Oil to toothbrush with baking soda; the soda is more effective than fluoride and hardens tooth enamel. Swish with Tea Tree Oil mixture twice daily, and swish for 3-5 minutes whenever possible; look for Tea Tree Oil dental floss in health stores. Also rub a few drops of pure Tea Tree Oil into the gums using a cotton swab, and massage.

TOOTHACHE

Supplies: Tea Tree Oil, aloe vera gel and mouthwash.

Remedy: Rinse teeth with gargle mixture, adding 3-5 drops of Tea Tree Oil to a mouthwash. You can also apply Tea Tree Oil along with a small amount of aloe vera gel directly onto infected tooth.

TOOTHBRUSH CARE

Supplies: Tea Tree Oil.

Remedy: Once or twice a week, apply a couple of drops of Tea Tree Oil to your toothbrush to help remove any bacteria.

NOTE: It is advisable not to use peroxide as it disturbs the oral flora; Tea Tree Oil does not do this.

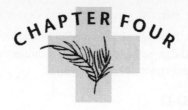

Throat and Chest

BRONCHIAL CONGESTION/BRONCHITIS

Condition: Bronchitis is an inflammation of the membrane that lines the air passages and bronchial tubes. The main symptoms are cough and increased expectoration, with or without associated wheezing and shortness of breath.

Supplies: Tea Tree Oil, cloth, grapeseed oil and cream.

Remedy: Steam chest with a mixture of 5 drops of Tea Tree Oil on a warm, wet cloth applied to chest. Add 10-12 drops of Tea Tree Oil to a hot bath; soak. Massage the infected area with 3 drops of Tea Tree Oil added to a cream, or to an oil such as grapeseed.

EMPHYSEMA

Condition: Emphysema is a disease of the lungs and often coexists with bronchitis.

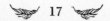 17

Supplies: Tea Tree Oil, cooking pot and vaporizer.

Remedy: Add 10 drops of Tea Tree Oil to a pot (4-6 cups) of hot water. Tent head, breathe steam for 10 minutes. Add 3-5 drops to a vaporizer, and steam for 5-10 minutes.

SORE THROAT

Condition: Sore throat or strep throat, is an inflammation of the throat and tonsils caused by bacteria.

Supplies: Tea Tree Oil, mouthwash, sea salt, cooking pot, towel, Tea Tree Oil/slippery elm lozenges and vaporizer.

Remedy: Add 3 drops of Tea Tree Oil to 4 ounces of warm water. You can add pinch of sea salt to the mixture and gargle 2-3 times daily. Tea Tree Oil mouthwash works also; or add 5 drops of Tea Tree Oil to 2 ounces of any mouthwash, and gargle. Put 10 drops of Tea Tree Oil into a pot of warm water (4-6 cups). Breathe in the vapors for 10 minutes, (tent your head and the pot with a towel). During the day, use Tea Tree Oil lozenges. A vaporizer in the bedroom, with 8 drops of Tea Tree Oil added, is also suggested.

> *NOTE: In Colorado, the air is always so dry. Thus my humidifier is always on. The added moisture, with Tea Tree Oil, is beneficial for my plants, animals and myself.*

COUGHS

Supplies: Tea Tree Oil, pot, vaporizer, slippery elm/Tea Tree Oil throat lozenges and grapeseed oil.

Remedy: Add 10 drops of Tea Tree Oil to 4-6 cups of warm water or 3-5 drops to a steam vaporizer, gently inhale. Some companies now produce Tea Tree Oil throat lozenges. These can be found in health stores.

THRUSH

Condition: A small oval budding yeast-like-fungus that resides in the throat, alimentary canal and the vagina. The condition is considered fungal and referred to as *Candida albicans*. When occurring in the mouth, it is commonly called Thrush.

Supplies: Tea Tree Oil and mouthwash.

Remedy: Add 5 drops of Tea Tree Oil to a cup of warm water, gargle 2-3 times daily. Add 5 drops of Tea Tree Oil to 1 ounce of mouthwash.

> *NOTE: Avoid any foods that contain yeast, bread, sugar, cheese and alcohol. Obtain an acidophilus powder from your health store.*

LARYNGITIS

Condition: Laryngitis is an inflammation of the larynx or voice box, usually associated with a common cold or overuse of the voice.

Supplies: Tea Tree Oil, mouthwash and slippery elm throat lozenges.

Remedy: Gargle as suggested for Thrush.

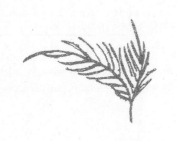

CHAPTER FIVE

Body

My mother developed rheumatoid arthritis when she was in her thirties; her situation was extreme. The doctor's prescription included cortisone, aspirin and gold shots. The problem was that the research didn't have a solution to the cause of her debilitating disease. There is now speculation that arthritis may be caused by a bacteria that attacks the urethra. Preventative measures include proper diet, exercise and stress management.

ARTHRITIS

Condition: Inflammation of joints; swelling, redness of the skin and impaired motion. Two types: 1) Osteo: chronic disease involving joints, especially weight-bearing joints; 2) Rheumatoid: chronic disease characterized by inflammatory changes in joints that may result in crippling.

Supplies: Tea Tree Oil, grapeseed or jojoba oil.

Remedy: For swelling, apply a flannel compress

> I've had arthritis for several years and find I get the greatest relief by applying Tea Tree Oil to the affected joint.
> *F.B. Carlsbad, CA*

21

with several drops of Tea Tree Oil and a clay poultice directly to affected area. A bath soak with 10 drops of the oil is also soothing.

Massage oil: Add 40 drops of Tea Tree Oil to 2 ounces of jojoba or grapeseed oil; massage into affected areas 2-3 times daily.

BRUISES

Supplies: Tea Tree Oil, arnica and comfrey.

Remedy: If swelling occurs, hold ice on bruised area for several minutes, then apply Tea Tree Oil twice daily, massage in well. Add several drops of Tea Tree Oil to an arnica or comfrey salve (see *Salve Recipes*, page 65). Apply daily. A cold compress over the salve helps.

BURNS (MINOR)

Condition: Reddening of the skin and blisters may occur.

Supplies: Tea Tree Oil, ice and salve.

Remedy: For reddening of the skin and possible blisters. Immediately wash area with ice water for one to two minutes. Apply several drops of oil on burned area, massage in well; alternate application of 100% Tea Tree Oil with ice water for up to one hour, depending on

In the early days of bush oil production, "cutters" were faced with hordes of wasps and hundreds of snakes, which hunted for frogs around the swamps. One distiller was badly burned on his arms, legs, back, and buttocks when his still exploded. He spent three weeks in a hospital and emerged with little or no scarring, which he claimed was because it was the Tea Tree Oil steam that burned him and the Tea Tree Oil steam that cured him!

severity of burn. Continue to massage Tea Tree Oil into burn twice daily for 3-4 days. This treatment will help to keep blistering and infection from occurring.

BURN SALVE: 5 oz. raw, unpasteurized honey mixed with 1 oz. Tea Tree Oil and 1 teaspoon grapefruit seed extract.

(Source: Puotinen, C.J. Natures Antiseptics: Tea Tree Oil and Grapefruit Seed Extract. New Canaan, CT; Keats Publishing, Inc., 1997).

DERMATITIS

Condition: This is an inflammation or irritation of the skin. The symptoms include itching, burning, redness, blistering, or edema (swelling).

Supplies: Tea Tree Oil, grapeseed oil, carrot oil, jojoba and Tea Tree Oil soap.

Remedy: For small areas, massage 5 drops of Tea Tree Oil into area; large areas: 10-20 drops of Tea Tree Oil into 1/4 cup of grapeseed oil. You may also add 10 drops of carrot or jojoba oil. Shake well. Massage this mixture in areas that have been exposed to water to help moisturize the skin. Apply twice a day. It is useful to wash with Tea Tree Oil soap.

Research: In 1991, Dr. Alvin Shemash, a family practitioner, and William Mayo, Ph.D., tested fifty patients with various skin problems. The purpose was to test and confirm the efficacy and safety of high quality Tea Tree Oil. The four patients with dermatitis and eczema were cured or showed remarkable improvement of their conditions. In this case, both Tea Tree Oil and a Tea Tree Oil cream were used.

ECZEMA

Condition: A non-contagious skin disorder that is characterized by itching skin on which scaly, red patches, as well as tiny, fluid-filled blisters, may appear.

Remedy: Make sure skin area is dry. Follow instructions for dermatitis.

HIVES

Condition: Reaction to allergies to foods, plants, chemicals or animals.

Supplies: Tea Tree Oil, witch hazel and Tea Tree Oil soap.

Remedy: Massage a few drops of Tea Tree Oil into affected area. For larger areas, make up a solution of 2 ounces of witch hazel to 15 drops of Tea Tree Oil. Wash with Tea Tree Oil soap.

MINOR CUTS AND ABRASIONS

Supplies: Tea Tree Oil, aloe vera gel and lavender oil.

Remedy: Clean area well, wash with Tea Tree soap. Apply a few drops of pure Tea Tree Oil to area with a dab of aloe vera gel and 2 drops of lavender oil. Apply twice daily; or you can make up a Tea Tree Oil salve instead.

I use Tea Tree Oil on all cuts, burns and most all my minor injuries. I call it the miracle oil and highly recommend it to all my friends. It heals very quickly.

P.M., Jessieville, AR

Salve: Make using calendula. (*see Salve Recipes*, page 65)

MUSCLE ACHES

Supplies: Tea Tree Oil, grapeseed oil and Tiger Balm®.

Remedy: Massage Tea Tree Oil into area; or warm 15 drops of Tea Tree, added to 1 ounce of grapeseed oil and massage in well. Bathe in warm water, with 10 drops of pure Tea Tree Oil added. After bath, add 2-3 drops of Tea Tree Oil to 1 ounce of Tiger Balm® (I prefer the red brand, it goes into sore muscles quite effectively).

PSORIASIS

Supplies: Tea Tree Oil, sea salt and evening primrose oil.

Remedy: Add 10 drops of Tea Tree Oil and one cup sea salt to bath water. (I buy 50 pound bags of sea salt from my local food co-op). For moisturizing, add 20 drops of Tea Tree Oil to 1 ounce of grapeseed oil; you may also add 10 drops of primrose or jojoba oil. Shake and massage in well.

RINGWORM

Condition: Superficial contagious infections caused by fungi that invade only dead tissues of the skin. Lesions with scaling and a slightly raised border. Easily transmitted in public places such as swimming pools and locker rooms.

Supplies: Tea Tree Oil.

Remedy: Apply Tea Tree Oil to area. Repeat twice daily.

RINGWORM OF SCALP *(TINEA CAPITAS)*

Supplies: Tea Tree Oil, shampoo and jojoba oil.

Remedy: Apply a few drops of Tea Tree Oil directly to affected area. Add 40 drops of Tea Tree Oil to 2 ounces of shampoo, and mix well. Use regularly until condition improves.

RINGWORM OF SKIN (*TINEA CORPORIS*)

Remedy: Add 30 drops of Tea Tree Oil to 1 ounce jojoba oil or aloe vera gel. Apply often. You may double this amount for larger areas. This remedy may also apply for treatment of Ringworm of Nails (*Tinea ungium*).

> *WARNING: Never use pure Tea Tree Oil on babies or young children. Always dilute with lotion or oil.*

WARTS

Condition: Warts are a form of viral infection. The most common warts are small, lumps that can grow anywhere on the skin, but most typically appear on the hands.

Supplies: Tea Tree Oil.

Remedy: Apply several drops of Tea Tree Oil to the wart. Keep area dry. May take several weeks to dissolve wart, depending upon condition.

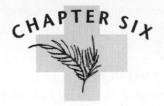

CHAPTER SIX

Legs & Feet

ATHLETES FOOT *(TINEA)*

Condition: Athlete's foot is caused by a fungus and is often accompanied by itching, burning and stinging.

Supplies: Tea Tree Oil, soap and olive oil.

Remedy: Wash feet with an anti-fungal soap and dry thoroughly. Apply pure Tea Tree Oil (or 10 drops of Tea Tree Oil mixed with 1/2 ounce of olive oil) onto and between toes. May also soak toes with 5 drops of Tea Tree Oil in a small bowl of water. Dry feet and apply Tea Tree Oil lotion into affected area.

> Tea Tree Oil is the best treatment I know for fungal infections of the skin (athlete's foot, ringworm, jock itch). It will also clear up fungal infections of the toenails, and fingernails, a condition notoriously resistant to treatment, even by strong systemic antibiotics.
>
> *Andrew Weil, M.D.*
> Natural Health, Natural Medicine

BLISTERS

Supplies: Tea Tree Oil, bandage and salve.

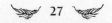

Remedy: Cleanse area gently with soap and water. Apply 2-3 drops of Tea Tree Oil onto area. Apply a Tea Tree Oil salve. Use Tea Tree Oil or salve twice daily.

CORNS AND CALLUSES

Condition: Corns taper into the skin like an inverted cone and are painful due to pressure on the nerve endings. A callus is an area of hardened and thickened skin, and is not usually painful.

Supplies: Tea Tree Oil, bandage, grapeseed oil, olive oil, cotton swabs and tweezers.

Remedy: Apply Tea Tree Oil using a cotton swab directly onto corn. Apply a mixture of 10 drops of Tea Tree Oil mixed into 1 teaspoon of grapeseed oil, and massage into the area well. A foot soak is useful; to a small basin of warm water, add 5 drops of a mixture of Tea Tree Oil, 1/2 ounce grapeseed oil or olive oil; soak for 5 minutes. This Tea Tree Oil mixture can be used directly on the area twice daily. When the corn becomes soft, remove with tweezers, apply 1-2 drops of Tea Tree Oil and cover with a bandage. Apply 2-3 times daily. A moisturizing lotion (see *Leg Ulcers,* page 29) applied directly into affected area also helps to soften the corns and calluses.

DIABETIC GANGRENE

Research: A study completed by Dr. Jill Fogarty, at Royal North Shore Hospital in Sydney, used hand and body lotion containing a 5% solution of Tea Tree Oil. The purpose of the study was to compare the skin on the legs of diabetic and geriatric patients. The 70 people in the study suffered from dry skin and or diabetes.

The cream was applied for a period of 25-26 days, on one leg only; dry skin became much softer, cracks healed and disappeared.

In 1936, *The Medical Journal of Australia* reported that Tea Tree Oil successfully treated diabetic gangrene.

Supplies: Tea Tree Oil, lotion.

Remedy: Blend 45 drops of Tea Tree Oil into 1/2 ounce of a lotion. Massage into affected area.

GOUT

Condition: Similar condition to arthritis; inflammation of joints, toes; swelling, redness of skin; diet high in protein may aggravate the condition.

Supplies and Remedy: See *Arthritis,* page 21

LEG ULCERS

Condition: An open, infected sore.

Supplies: Tea Tree Oil and grapeseed oil.

Remedy: Massage a few drops of pure Tea Tree Oil into affected area on the legs 2-3 times daily. Soak the ulcer in a bowl of warm water, to which 5 drops of Tea Tree Oil has been added.

Massage Moisturizing Lotion: Add 30 drops of pure Tea Tree Oil into 1 ounce of grapeseed oil, shake well.

> *NOTE: If irritation occurs, discontinue use of pure Tea Tree Oil and use Tea Tree Oil moisturizing lotion instead, once or twice a day.*

PLANTAR WARTS *(VERUCCAE PLANTARIS)*

Condition: Common, contagious, epithelical tumors caused by at least 60 types of human papillomavirus (HPV). Since the warts appear on the soles of the feet they can be painful and difficult to treat. It's been noted that people with suppressed immune systems are more susceptible to this condition.

Supplies: Tea Tree Oil, myrrh and bandage.

Remedy: Apply Tea Tree Oil to affected area 2-3 times daily. Equal amounts of Tea Tree Oil and myrrh applied and covered with a bandage will help soften the warts, thus making them easier to remove with a sterilized needle.

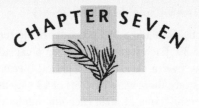

Personal Hygiene

NOTE; Many of these suggested uses should be applied with care. If any of the symptoms do not subside within a reasonable amount of time, consult your health practitioner.

BLADDER INFECTION *(CYSTITIS)*

Condition: Cystitis is an inflammation of the wall and lining of the urinary bladder, often due to bacterial infection but sometimes caused by abrasion from microcrystals of calcium phosphate in urine.

Supplies: Tea Tree Oil and distilled water.

Remedy: For hygiene purposes, it is important to keep the urethra cleaned. Prepare a mild solution of 3 drops of pure Tea Tree Oil, mixed into 4 ounces of purified or distilled water. Use this solution to wash the area thoroughly. Bathe, adding 10 drops of the pure Tea Tree Oil into the tub water.

Research: Dr Belaiche did a second study on 26 female patients, of average age 39. Each woman was given a capsule of Tea Tree Oil once a day over a three- month period. Because this was a double-blind study, there were two lots of 13 patients each. Lot A was given 24 milligrams of *Melaleuca alternifolia* (Tea Tree Oil) daily - 3 doses of 8 milligrams before main meals. Lot B received a placebo. After 6 months, Lot B showed no improvement, while Lot A, 7 (out of 13) were cured.

(Source: Phytotherapie, September 1985. No 115, pp. 9-11).

HEMORRHOIDS

Condition: Hemorrhoids, or piles, are tender, painful swellings. They tend to occur in pregnant women and in persons with chronic constipation, and are believed to be a result of diets low in fiber.

Supplies: Tea Tree Oil, witch hazel and comfrey.

> **From this first clinical approach, it is apparent that the essential oil of Melaleuca alternifolia is effectively efficient for the treatment of chronic colibacilli cystitis.**
> *Dr. Paul Belaiche*

Remedy: Apply several drops of Tea Tree Oil directly onto affected area; soak in tub using 10 drops of Tea Tree Oil in water. Also add 10 drops of Tea Tree Oil to a comfrey salve ointment; apply twice daily.

Make a cold compress using 2 ounces of witch hazel and 1 tablespoon Tea Tree Oil. Apply for 10 minutes.

For extreme swelling, a Tea Tree Oil suppository can be used. (See *Ovarian Cysts*, page 33)

HERPES LESIONS *(SIMPLEX TYPE II)*

Condition: Contagious viral condition. Easily transmitted between people.

Supplies: Tea Tree Oil, vitamin E and aloe vera gel.

Remedy: Mix 5 drops of pure Tea Tree Oil with 1 capsule of Vitamin E. Apply twice daily. If irritation occurs discontinue use. Soak in a bath adding 10 drops of Tea Tree Oil; Sitz bath: 25 drops of Tea Tree Oil and 1 teaspoon aloe gel, soak.

JOCK ITCH *(TINEA CRURIS)*

Condition: A fungal infection of male groin area and fingernails.

Supplies: Tea tree oil, anti-fungal soap, grapeseed oil, carrot oil and alcohol (Everclear or vodka is preferrable to isopropyl).

Remedy: Twice daily rub several drops of tea tree oil on affected area. If this is too strong, use a solution of 1/2 ounce alcohol add 1 ounce of Tea Tree Oil; mix and apply.

Massage Oil: Add 15 drops of tea tree oil to 1/2 ounce grapeseed oil. A 10% solution of carrot oil can be added. Apply 2 times daily.

> After using Tea Tree Oil in my busy herbalist/naturopath practice.. (it) works really well with the herpes simplex blisters.. it replaces antibiotic powders.
>
> *Herbal Practitioner, Australia*

OVARIAN CYSTS

Supplies: Tea Tree Oil, suppositories and tampon.

Remedy: Obtain Tea Tree Oil suppositories if possible through you health store; insert. The suppository will melt and help to reduce the cysts. If suppositories are not available, use a Tea Tree Oil saturated tampon (3-5 drops of Tea Tree Oil) and insert for 24 hours. May be used daily; if symptoms don't change, consult your physician.

VAGINITIS

Condition: Usually caused by a yeast infection, *Candida albicans*. Several situations may result in an outbreak of yeast in the body. Poor nutrition, lack of adequate water consumption, sweating and wearing tight clothing all may contribute to an outbreak of yeast. The areas which may be affected are the mouth, vagina, buttocks, and between the breasts.

Supplies: Tea Tree Oil, tampon and douche bag.

Remedy: Douche with 8-10 drops of pure Tea Tree Oil mixed into 1 pint of distilled or purified water. Treatment can be done daily until symptoms subside or disappear. Between douching, saturate a tampon with several drops of Tea Tree Oil and insert, leave in 24 hours. A light sensation may be felt. Add 10 drops of pure Tea Tree Oil to a tub of warm water; soak for 20 minutes.

Research: In 1985, Dr Paul Belaiche from the University of Paris, conducted a study on patients with thrush, a vaginal infection of *Candida albicans*. His study focused on 28 patients using a Tea Tree Oil suppository inserted into the vagina every evening. Upon examination 30 days later, 21 out of 28 patients showed complete recovery. Dr. Belaiche felt Tea Tree Oil to be very effective, less irritating than other essential oils, and easily tolerated by vaginal membranes.

(Source: Phtotherapie, Vol 15, 1985)

The Wigan Hospital in England found Tea Tree Oil to be more effective in treating oral candidiasis than the drug Fluconazole for Yeast Infections.

(Source: International Journal of Aromatherapy 1994,Vol.5).

WAXING BIKINI AREA/LEGS

Supplies: Tea Tree Oil, Tea Tree Oil lotion and witch hazel.

Remedy: Before waxing apply 3-5 drops of Tea Tree Oil to area. Allow to dry; after treatment apply Tea Tree Oil again and follow up with Tea Tree Oil lotion; repeat 2 times same day. Redness and swelling should subside within 24 hours. Helps to eliminate ingrown hairs. For a soothing and nourishing leg toner: combine 10 drops of pure Tea Tree Oil with equal parts of water and witch hazel (4 ounces each).

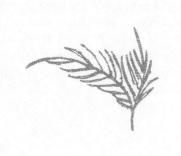

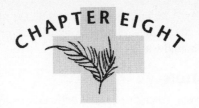

CHAPTER EIGHT

Beauty Care

Tea Tree Oil has been known to penetrate into the skin's cellular level. The antiseptic benefits of Tea Tree Oil help to clear up blemishes and leave the skin feeling clean. Tea Tree Oil skin cream helps oxygenate skin cells, while aiding in the repair of damage caused by sun, acne, dryness, fungus, and other various skin ailments.

There are a number of Tea Tree Oil skin and bodycare products available through beauty suppliers, health stores, and mainstream outlets such as sunscreen, massage oil, soap, antiseptics, deodorants, acne cream, and other creams and lotions. You may purchase these products or add Tea Tree Oil to your own creams and lotions. (see Chapter 2, *Face*).

ACNE MASK:

Supplies: Tea Tree Oil, neroli, rosemary or thyme oil and clay.

Remedy: Add 1-4 drops of neroli, rosemary or thyme oil to a small amount of clay. Add 5 drops of Tea Tree Oil. Let mask sit on face for less than 20 minutes; remove mask with warm water; splash 20 times with cold water.

BODY LOTION

There are several splendid, natural body lotions that can be purchased through health spas, body care shops and health food stores. Stay away from artificial additives, petroleum based products (including mineral oil and Vaseline), and any ingredients that you cannot pronounce, let alone understand the meaning of!

Remedy: Find a lotion that feels moisturizing and good to your skin, add 15 drops of Tea Tree Oil to the lotion, shake well. Apply lotion immediately after a shower; massage into feet, ankles, legs, abdomen, buttocks and arms, using your fingers to work the lotion into your skin.

BODY SMOOTHER

The skin is the largest organ of our body. Maintaining it with massage, dry-brushing, diet, exercise and nutrients will provide us with a supple and rosy skin tone.

DRY BRUSHING

Supplies: Natural bristle brush.

Remedy: Before bath or shower, brush beginning at toes toward your heart. Use long sweeping motions. Brush legs and abdomen, with upward motion on arms. Apply a few drops of Tea Tree Oil to a squeeze of aloe vera gel, and massage into face and neck. This quick treatment will hydrate the skin while bathing. Shower and finish with cold water to close pores and invigorate the body. Using a terry towel, buff your skin dry.

DRY SKIN

Supplies: Tea Tree Oil, neroli and carrot seed oil.

Remedy: Add 1-4 drops of neroli and carrot seed oil with 5 drops of Tea Tree Oil to a small container of yogurt or fruits, such as papaya with honey. Apply to dry skin. Leave on for 20 minutes, rinse thoroughly.

> *NOTE: It is advisable not to use grapeseed oil as a carrier oil for the face area, since it is a heavy oil and can clog the facial skin.*

Tea Tree Oil is the best treatment I know for fungal infections of the skin. It will also clear up fungal infections of the toenails and fingernails, a condition notoriously resistant to treatment, even by strong systemic antibiotics. You just paint the oil on affected area two to three times a day.

Andrew Weil, M.D.
Natural Health, Natural Medicine

FACIAL MASK - OILY SKIN

Supplies: Tea Tree Oil, lavender oil and clay.

Remedy: Mix 1-4 drops of lavender oil into clay, and add 5 drops of Tea Tree Oil. Allow mask to sit for less than 20 minutes. Rinse by taking a warm, wet washcloth, pressing gently to remove mask thoroughly; then rinse face with 20 splashes of cold water to close the pores and revitalize the skin.

NAIL SOAK

Supplies: Tea Tree Oil, nail file, lotion, olive oil and almond oil.

Remedy: Remove polish, smooth nail surface, shape nails. Warm a Tea Tree Oil hand and body lotion; or a blend of 10 drops pure Tea Tree Oil and 2 tablespoons olive or almond oil. Soak nails for 5 minutes. Massage lotion around nailbeds and fingers twice daily. Tissue off excess. Do twice daily until infection clears.

NAIL STAINS

Supplies: Tea Tree Oil and iodine.

Remedy: Buff the nail with iodine and a few drops of Tea Tree Oil. Buff off the milky white to remove all the stain from the nail.

NAIL INFECTIONS *(PERIONYCHIA)*

There have been horror stories about women refusing to treat their nail fungus, asking the manicurist to cut back the infected nail and slap another nail on top. The following applications will keep fungus away.

Supplies: Tea Tree Oil, olive oil, almond oil and wheat germ oil.

Remedy: Apply pure Tea Tree Oil to affected area and around cuticles, massage in well. Do not rinse off. Affected area can be soaked for 5 minutes daily with 10 drops of Tea Tree Oil to 2 tablespoons of olive, almond oil or wheat germ oil.

CHAPTER NINE

Home Care & On The Road

Homes and office work spaces are exposed to various viruses, microorganisms and radon gas; allergic responses to synthetic household goods and carpets, pet hair, cleaning solvents, and paint, (to name a few) are common. Offices, hospitals, airplanes and venting systems are poorly designed. Masses of people arrive and depart from airports everyday. Unhealthy microorganisms are rampant. "If you want to get sick, go to a hospital," has become a coined phrase.

Viruses and bacteria are everywhere. In most modern buildings there are few windows that provide any circulation of fresh air. Lack of green plants reduces fresh oxygen supplies. All of these situations create conditions that encourage illness. The following uses for Tea Tree Oil at home, in care centers, offices, and while traveling will improve our ability to sustain good health, while exposed to ever-increasing unhealthy environments.

SECTION I - HOUSEHOLD CLEANING

AUTHOR'S NOTES

Disinfectant/ Cleanser: As we were completing this edition, a bulletin was sent to my email address announcing the possible dangers of yet another mass market product that is advertised as "anti-bacterial." The products are yellow sponges with green plastic fibers, and anti-bacterial dish and hand soaps. The anti-bacterialchemical is called *triclosan,* a derivative of the systemic pesticide/herbicide, 2-4-D, more popularly known as *Agent Orange*. The warning in small letters states, that the fungicide cannot be washed from the sponge even if it is placed in a dishwasher, which now spreads it to kitchen utensils, pots, dishes and glassware. There are several reports that aquarium tanks were cleaned using one of these sponges, and within 5 hours after filling the tank, all of the tropical fish died. There is a warning that states, "Not for use in aquariums. Keep away from other pets."

A much safer alternative is to purchase disinfectant household cleaners, laundry detergents and dish-washing formulas from Tea Tree Oil manufacturers. Tea Tree Oil acts as a powerful antiseptic, proven to be 10-13 times stronger than the number-one chemical antiseptic, carbolic acid. Thus cleaning and washing with Tea Tree Oil helps provide a naturally safe environment for the entire family.

Essential Oil: Household cleaners, add 10-15 drops Tea Tree Oil.

Food Grade Hydrogen Peroxide: To make a 3% solution: purchase 35% food grade hydrogen peroxide (H_2O_2) at your health food store. Mix one ounce of 35% into 11 ounces of distilled water. This makes 3/4 pint of 3% Hydrogen Peroxide.

CAUTION: *When handling H_2O_2 avoid any contact with eyes. If it comes in contact with skin, wash immediately with warm water. Do not keep in refrigerator where it can be mistaken for water. Keep out of reach of children.*

ALICE'S WONDER SPRAY™

Supplies: Liquid soap or detergent, white distilled vinegar, borax, purified water, essential oil, 16 ounce trigger spray bottle.

Recipe: Mix 2 tbsp. of vinegar with 1 tsp. borax. Fill the rest of the bottle with very hot water. Shake until the borax is dissolved. Add 1/4 cup of liquid soap, or 1/8 cup of liquid detergent. To scent, add 10-15 drops of an essential oil.

Special notes: Because minerals in the water inhibit cleaning, it's best to use purified or distilled water. It's also important to dissolve the borax in hot water so that it doesn't clog the spray nozzle. Do not mix the soap and vinegar directly together, because the soap will clump up. Instead, mix the vinegar, borax and water first and then add the soap last. Borax is an eye irritant and can be harmful if swallowed,

WARNING: Keep out of reach of children.

How to use: Spray and wipe. Use as you would any other all-purpose household cleaner. Use on refrigerator, walls, tile, shower, shelves and toilets. Because it is not as chemically powerful as commercial cleaners, give it a little more time to work on difficult stains. One batch will last 6 months.

(Source: Clean House, Clean Planet by Karen Logan, Pocket Books. Reference: Excerpt by permission from Co-op America, 1612 K St. NW, Ste. 600, Washington, DC 20077-2573, (800) 584-7336, www.coopamerica.org).

CHEMICALS IN CLEANING PRODUCTS

To "demystify" which cleaning products are safe to use throughout your home/work space; and to provide a cleaner and environmentally safer way to clean, here is a list of substances found in conventional household cleaners.

Glycol: Ether, naphtha, kerosene - neuro-toxins and central nervous system depressants that can cause confusion, headaches, lack of concentration, and symptoms of mental illness.

Sodium Bromide: May cause confusion.

Morpholine: Very toxic, liver and kidney poison.

Bleach, chlorinated phosphates: Can form toxic, carcinogenic and mutagenic chlorinate compounds (endocrine disrupters like DDT) in the environment.

EDTA: Binds with heavy metals in lakes and streams and activates these metals.

Petroleum-based products: Nonrenewable resource, slow to break down in the environment.

Complex phosphates: Cause algae bloom.

(Sources: Clean and Green by Annie Berthold-Bond, 1994, Ceres Press, (914) 679-5573; Clean House, Clean Planet. Co-op America's Real Money, Spring 1999 Vol.1 No2. Reference: Excerpt by permission from Co-op America, 1612 K St. NW, Ste. 600, Washington, DC 20077-2573, (800) 584-7336, www.coopamerica.org).

DISHWASHERS

Use 1 tbsp. 20 Mule Team Borax®, 3-5 drops of Tea Tree Oil-2 ounces of 3% food grade hydrogen peroxide, with a biodegradable natural dishwashing detergent.

HOUSEHOLD CLEANING SOLUTION

Supplies: Tea Tree Oil and washing soda.

Remedy: Add 15 drops of Tea Tree Oil to 1 quart of water, add 1/2 cups of washing soda, and 1/4 cup of 190 proof vodka or everclear. This simple formula will clean your entire house. It is non-carcinogenic and will deodorize and leave your home free of bacteria, germs and mold.

PLANTS

Research: In an antiviral study, Tea Tree Oil was applied to Nicotinia glutinosa plants, which were then inoculated with tobacco virus. Tea Tree Oil reduced the number of virus-induced lesions on the plants.

To deter insects, molds and fungus from plants, the following suggestions are beneficial:

Supplies: Tea Tree Oil, mister, food grade hydrogen peroxide 35%.

Remedy: To a 32-oz. bottle of water, add 20 drops of Tea Tree Oil and 16 drops of hydrogen peroxide. Mix well. Mist plants; do not wipe off. Use for a week. If plants are not responding, discontinue use.

WASHING MACHINES

Use 20 Mule Team Borax® and Washing Soda®; following instructions on box , add 20 drops of Tea Tree Oil for each load; add 6 ounces of 3% food grade hydrogen peroxide (to replace bleach).

SECTION II - NURSING HOME CARE

BEDSORES

Supplies: Tea Tree Oil and almond or olive oil.

Remedy: For a person in the house or nursing home who is bed-ridden. A small application of Tea Tree Oil will help to soothe and eliminate bedsores. Massage 5 drops of Tea Tree Oil mixed with 1 tablespoon of almond or olive oil onto affected parts of the body. Repeat as required.

HAND DISINFECTANT

Hands of staff members in hospitals and nursing facilities remain the main mode for transmission of cross-infections. *The anti-microbial activity of Tea Tree Oil lends itself as a hygienic hand disinfectant. There are no apparent dermatological problems with constant use of Tea Tree disinfectant soaps as with other products.*

Research: In a recent study, in the Journal of Hospital Infections, researchers said that 0.5 percent Tea Tree Oil killed 60 strains of antibiotic-resistant *Staph aureus*, bacteria that cause secondary infections in hospitals and long-term care facilities.

(Source: 1) Susceptibility of transient and commensal skin flora to the essential oil of Melaleuca alternifolia (Tea Tree Oil). Hammer, Carson, Riley; Department of Microbiology, Nedlands, Western Australia, 1996. 2) Natural Foods Merchandiser, February 1999).

HUMIDIFIER

Adding 10 drops of Tea Tree Oil to the humidifier will clean the air and leave it smelling fresh. Periodically, I clean out my humidifier in a tub of water in which 10 drops of Tea Tree Oil have been added, scrub the tank well, change the filter, and refill the tank. It's lovely to add 2-3 drops of another fragrant essential oil. One of my favorites is lavender.

MOOD/MEMORY PICK-ME-UPPER

A massage, facial and mister with 2 drops of Tea Tree Oil lemon, rosemary or chamomile essential oils and distilled water can elevate moods and energize the brain.

ROOM FRESHENER

Supplies: Tea Tree Oil, spray bottle and lavender oil.

Remedy: Add 10 drops of Tea Tree Oil to a spray bottle, add 3 drops of lavender. Mist rooms. If traveling, add several drops of Tea Tree Oil to the hotel room venting system or carry a purse size mister.

VAPORIZER

Add 10 drops of Tea Tree Oil to the water; leave in room to help alleviate stuffiness, allergies, headaches and flu symptoms. Another method which was suggested earlier in the book is to heat up a pot of water, add several drops of Tea Tree Oil, remove pot from stove, using a towel tent the patient, and breathe in the vapors for 10 minutes.

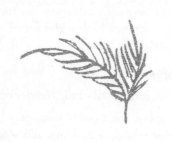

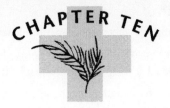

CHAPTER TEN

Aromatherapy

Aromatherapy is the use of essential oils, which may stimulate extraordinary individual changes on the physical, emotional, mental, or spiritual levels. A pure essential oil is the highly concentrated essence of a plant from the root, bark, flower and/or leaf. Essential oils can be mixed with a carrier oil such as jojoba, and blended into massage lotions, bath oils, cosmetics, perfumes, facial masks, compresses, and used in saunas and diffusers.

Tea Tree Oil is discussed in Robert Tisserand's books, *Aromatherapy for Everyone* and *The Art of Aromatherapy*, available through book and health stores.

Warning: Dilute all essential oils; they are concentrated and can be irritating to the skin. Do not take internally.

BATH SALTS

Excellent for muscle aches and general relaxation.

Supplies: 1 cup Epsom salts, 1/2 cup Borax, 1/2 cup sea salt, 1/2 cup baking soda 1/2 teaspoon of rosemary oil.

Remedy: Draw a bath, add 10 drops of Tea Tree Oil and the bath salts and oil (above).

DEEP HAIR CONDITIONER

Supplies: Mix 1 drop Tea Tree Oil, 1 beaten egg and 1 tbsp. carrier oil (jojoba or olive).

Remedy: Wash hair, apply conditioner for 5-10 minutes, rinse.

DEODORIZER

Add 10-20 drops of Tea Tree Oil into a mister, diffuser, humidifier or vaporizer to clean and sanitize the air.

Tea Tree Oil definitely can be added to a list of other fine essential oils as a great contribution to Aromatherapy. Remember to shop for only the pure essential oils as there are many Aromatherapy products that have perfumes and other artificial scents added. Store pure Tea Tree Oil in amber glass bottles to preserve its essence and integrity. Keep away from heat and light; store in a cool place. When mixing small amounts of Tea Tree Oil into other lotions, plastics are suitable.

DRY SKIN

Add 6 drops of Tea Tree Oil, vetivert and sandalwood oil into 1 ounce of carrier oil such as carrot seed or sweet almond.

HAIR RINSE - FOR SCALP

Add 2-3 drops of Tea Tree Oil into 32 fluid ounces of water.

MASSAGE

By combining 5-10 drops of Tea Tree Oil with other massage oils, the skin will receive relief from sore muscles and leave the body refreshed, clean and healthy.

PERFUME BODY MIST

Add 2 drops of Tea Tree Oil and 2 drops of pure rose oil, into one teaspoon of jojoba oil.

VAPORIZER

By adding several drops of Tea Tree Oil to a vaporizer and placing it in a room where an ill person is resting, the mist will help deodorize and clean the air. The person will benefit as well by breathing the vapors. When used in a diffuser (*small Aromatherapy machine*), the aroma is like sitting in a grove of Tea Trees in the Australian bush!

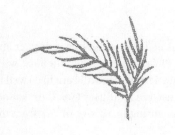

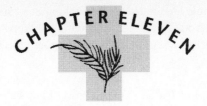

Baby & Child Care

God's special angels on earth ~
It is always recommended and important to remember that babies and children have very sensitive skin. It is best for them to mix Tea Tree Oil with quality cold-pressed oil.

CHICKEN POX *(HERPES ZOSTER)*

Condition: A highly contagious virus (also affiliated with outbreaks of shingles).

Supplies: Tea Tree Oil, calamine lotion, vaporizer, oatmeal and lavender.

Remedy: Use the sug-

I had chicken pox for two weeks, and the itching was incredible... I used calamine lotion, soaked a couple of times a day in oatmeal... I put Tea Tree Oil, 10 drops; lavender, 10 drops; and lemon, 5 drops - in 2 tablespoons of vegetable oil. I dabbed this mixture on the pox on my face a few times a day. My face healed faster than my body, and I have absolutely no scars on my face.

gested formula mentioned above. Soaking in a bathtub using the measles method is suggested, and adding 10 drops of Tea Tree Oil to the vaporizer reservoir will keep the room fresh and clean.

COLDS

Add 10 drops of Tea Tree Oil to a bowl of hot water or vaporizer. Leave vaporizer in baby's area overnight or whenever indicated. A small handkerchief sprinkled with Tea Tree Oil under baby's/child's pillow may help as well.

CRADLE CAP *(DERMATITIS)*

Condition: Cradle Cap - Dermatitis of a newborn, usually appearing on scalp, face, and head. Thick, yellowish crusted lesions will develop on the scalp and scaling will appear behind ears.

Supplies: Tea Tree Oil, olive oil and shampoo.

Remedy: Mix 5 drops of Tea Tree Oil with 2 tbsp. olive oil; rub into scalp, leave for 5 minutes; wash and rinse. Use a Tea Tree Oil shampoo mixture, being careful to keep out of child's eyes.

DIAPER CLEANSER

Remedy: Add 20 drops of Tea Tree Oil or a water miscible formula to each gallon of water. Stir and soak diapers overnight. (See *Water Miscible Mixtures,* page 67)

DIAPER RASH *(NAPPY RASH)*

Supplies: Tea Tree Oil, calendula and baby lotion.

Remedy: Add 5 drops of Tea Tree Oil to a calendula salve (see *Salve Recipes,* page 65). You may also add 10 drops to 1/4 cup of a natural baby lotion (found in health stores). Do not use petroleum based products. There are substitutes for Vaseline which do not contain petroleum.

NOTE: *Do not apply pure Tea Tree Oil to a baby's bottom.*

EARACHES/EAR INFECTIONS

Supplies: Tea Tree Oil, olive oil, dropper and cotton ball.

Remedy: Warm 5 drops of Tea Tree Oil with a teaspoon of olive oil. Trickle a small amount in ear. Apply as needed.

HEAT AND SKIN RASH

Supplies: Tea Tree Oil and calendula salve.

Remedy: Add 1-2 drops of Tea Tree Oil to a calendula salve (see *Salve Recipes*, page 65). Reapply as needed.

IMPETIGO STREPTOCOCCUS (OR *STAPHYLOCOCCUS BACTERIA*)

Condition: Highly contagious; pimples or blisters on neck, scalp and face.

Supplies: Tea Tree Oil and calamine lotion.

Remedy: Add 10 drops of Tea Tree Oil to 4 tbsp. of calamine lotion. Apply to infected areas 2-3 times daily. Add 5 drops of Tea Tree Oil to bath water.

INSECT BITES

Supplies: Tea Tree Oil, witch hazel and calamine lotion.

Remedy: Combine 2 tbsp. of witch hazel or calamine lotion and

5 drops of Tea Tree Oil; shake and apply 2-3 times daily. You may dab a couple of drops immediately on bitten area.

MEASLES *(RED MEASLES - RUBEOLA VIRUS)*

Condition: A highly contagious virus. The symptoms include, a high fever, red spots on skin, sensitivity to light, and sore throat often accompanied by a cough.

Supplies: Tea Tree Oil, vaporizer, witch hazel.

Remedy: One of my daughters at an earlier age ran high fevers. I would run a cool bath and sponge her down to help lower the fever. The same application can be done for measles: add 5 drops of Tea Tree Oil to a small amount of cool bath water, and sponge the child's body.

For older children you may apply a lotion mixing 2 ounces of witch hazel with 5 drops of Tea Tree Oil. Apply lotion with a cotton ball over affected areas.

Warning: Do not use on babies.

To alleviate cough and sore throat: you may use the steam inhaler; adding 5 drops of Tea Tree Oil to 4 cups of boiled water. Have the child inhale the vapors. A draped towel works or a paper bag in which the bottom has been cut out to make a tent.

Gargle with 2-4- ounces of warm water, a shake of sea salt and 3 drops of Tea Tree Oil.

To keep the child's room antiseptically clean, add 10 drops of Tea Tree Oil to the vaporizer's reservoir.

ROOM DEODORIZER AND DISINFECTANT

Supplies: Tea Tree Oil and diffuser.

Remedy: If you have a diffuser, add a few drops of Tea Tree Oil to freshen and clean the baby's area. A humidifier or vaporizer will work as well; adding five to ten drops of Tea Tree Oil to the water will add a wonderful mist to the baby's room.

SORE BREASTS *(FROM BREAST FEEDING)*

Supplies: Tea Tree Oil, Vitamin E and lotion.

Remedy: If breasts are sore, dry or cracked, massage a small amount of Tea Tree Oil lotion onto the area.

Make a soothing lotion: Add 10 drops of Tea Tree Oil to 1 teaspoon of Vitamin E, add to your favorite healthy lotion. Apply as needed.

TONSILLITIS

Condition: A virus and/or from Streptococcal bacteria.

My granddaughter has reoccurring bouts of tonsillitis. I have given her a small cup of warm water, added 3-4 drops of Tea Tree Oil and a shake of sea salt and had her gargle thoroughly at the back of her throat until the glass is empty. This has given her relief within a short amount of time. I suggested to my daughter to enhance her immune system by consulting with her practitioner.

Supplies: Tea Tree Oil and sea salt.

Remedy: Use the suggested gargle mentioned above. For soothing relief, rub a few drops of Tea Tree Oil on the outside of the throat area.

NOTE: Keep Tea Tree Oil stored in a place where younger children cannot reach.

Research: When my youngest daughter was less than 2 years old, she swallowed some lemon oil polish; she was taken to the hospital, and other than slight diarrhea, she was free of other symptoms. Children's Hospital in Seattle, Washington reported that a 17 month-old, ingested less than 10 ml (approximately 1/3 ounce) of 100% pure Tea Tree Oil. Approximately 10 minutes after the ingestion, the child became sleepy, appeared unsteady, and was unable to walk or sit. There was no difficulty in breathing. The child remained under observation and was free of symptoms within 3 hours. Clinical experience with ingestion of Tea Tree Oil is limited; however, a modest amount (unknown) may produce signs of toxicity.

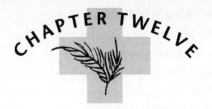

Outdoors & Camping

BLISTERS

Supplies: Tea Tree Oil and bandage.

Remedy: Put Tea Tree Oil directly on blister. Apply a sterile, non-stick bandage.

FIRE ANT BITES

I was introduced to Tea Tree Oil in 1985 after receiving a wicked bite from these ants, *(not the kind of relatives you welcome to your home)*!

Supplies: Tea Tree Oil salve. (see *Salve Recipes,* page 65)

Remedy: Cover area with salve. Do not open blister; doing so will release the formic acid, which dissolves skin.

INSECT BITES AND STINGS

Supplies: Tea Tree Oil, grapeseed oil, lotion, salve, calamine, peppermint oil and baking soda.

Remedy: Apply 2-3 drops of Tea Tree Oil to the bite. For larger areas, combine 5 drops of Tea Tree Oil to a cold-pressed oil such as grapeseed. I recommend this oil above others because it does not stain clothing and linens, as almond oil does. For children: mix 3-5 drops into a lotion, such as calamine. Shake well, apply 2-3 times daily. There are ways to remove the stinger if you do not have allergic reactions. Mix green clay, 2-3 drops of Tea Tree Oil and water to make a paste; cover the area, allow to dry and pull off. Usually the stinger will come out. To stop itch, mix 3-5 drops of Tea Tree Oil with a paste of peppermint oil and baking soda.

INSECT REPELLENT

Supplies: Tea Tree Oil and first aid lotion.

Remedy: Apply oil to exposed areas of the body to help ward off insects. Make your own insect repellent by adding 10-20 drops of Tea Tree Oil to citronella. Mix well. This is extremely useful for hiking, and camping.

LEECHES

Condition: A parasitical bloodsucking worm; resides in water.

Supplies: Tea Tree Oil, protective clothing.

Remedy: Hiking or camping outdoors, apply Tea Tree Oil to exposed areas. It is advisable to wear long sleeved shirts, socks and long pants while in the wilderness. Make up a Tea Tree spray in a small portable spray bottle, which can be carried in your backpack . Add 10 drops of Tea Tree Oil to a natural bug repellent, spray frequently. Inspect your body for leeches thoroughly. Once they are on, difficult to remove. Apply pure Tea Tree Oil directly onto leech site; allow 15 minutes to absorb; leech should remove itself.

POISON IVY/POISON OAK/POISON SUMAC

Supplies: Tea Tree Oil, oatmeal soap, baking soda, lavender and gauze bandage.

Remedy: Wash with oatmeal soap. Mix a paste of baking soda and 5-10 drops of Tea Tree Oil, spread over area. Keep blisters from breaking open by applying gauze. Apply the Tea Tree Oil paste 2-3 times daily. Soak in a bath with 10 drops of Tea Tree Oil and lavender oil added.

SANDFLEAS

Remedy: Follow the instructions for insect bites/stings and repellent.

SPLINTERS

Supplies: Tea Tree Oil, tweezers.

Remedy: Clean area thoroughly with an antiseptic soap, apply 2-3 drops of Tea Tree Oil to area. Try to remove with tweezers. For lodged splinter pieces, massage a couple more drops of the oil into area. In time, the pieces should become dislodged.

SPRAINS

I once had a bad sprain while trekking around the Costa Rican rainforest. Thank goodness I had my reliable Tea Tree Oil with me. After holding the area for 10 minutes (which helps to keep swelling down), I applied Tea Tree Oil to my ankle every day.

Supplies: Tea Tree Oil, arnica and gauze.

Remedy: ICE - Ice, Compress, Elevate *(first aid procedure)*. Apply arnica and several drops of Tea Tree Oil, wrap area with dry cloth or bandage. Rest with foot elevated for at least 20 minutes, repeat often during the day.

SUNBURN

Supplies: Tea Tree Oil, Tea Tree cream, Vitamin E oil, almond oil and avocado oil.

Remedy: High altitude is hard on the skin. Protect it with a moisturizing sun cream (leave out the PABA). Use a Tea Tree cream and/or mix a few drops of Tea Tree Oil with Vitamin E oil, almond or avocado oil. Apply twice daily.

> While vacationing in Santa Fe one summer I was unaware of how intense the sun could be at that altitude. As a result of lying by the swimming pool for part of an afternoon, I received a painful sunburn. For the next few days I soaked in a bath of Tea Tree Oil several times. The pain disappeared immediately and my skin never dried, cracked or peeled. I have never tried anything that worked so well.
> *D.E., OK*

TICKS

During my summer camp activities, hiking through the dense bush in the Adirondack Mountains of N.Y., ticks were a common occurrence. Today, Lyme's Disease is associated with tick fever.

Supplies: Tea Tree Oil, tweezers.

Remedy: Apply Tea Tree Oil directly to the site; within a short time, if the tick has not backed out of the skin, use tweezers to extract it. If cold-like symptoms or a ring-like pattern appear around the area, consult with your physician.

LETTER FROM A CAMPER ON USE OF TEA TREE OIL

As an avid rafter and camper, I have found Australian Tea Tree Oil to be indispensable on my many yearly outings. Not only do I use it for the typical scrapes, sunburns, muscle soreness, and abrasions that go along with this lifestyle, I also use it for personal hygiene as well.

Any person who spends time camping, etc. with a group of people, is aware of the absolute necessity of antiseptic measures ritual under these circumstances. Everyone has a responsibility not only to themselves, but also to the rest of the group, not to be a source of contamination. We all share a portable toilet, and we all take turns cooking.

If proper care is not taken in the area of personal cleanliness everyone can suffer, and the trip can be ruined. Therefore it is imperative that each time one uses the toilet, one immediately uses an antibacterial handwash. I add 15-20 drops of Tea Tree Oil to each ounce of liquid soap, such as Dr. Bronner's, and put it by the portable commode that is required when camping in National Forests. In this concentration it is known to kill 99% of bacteria on contact, and is ENVIRONMENTALLY SAFE to rivers, streams, fauna and flora.

Long ago I quit using store-bought antibacterial soaps. I just recently found out that their active ingredient was a component of **Agent Orange**! Also, I never felt comfortable about the use of chlorine as a disinfectant in dish water, as the typical protocol calls for dumping this water back into the river. I have found that using Tea Tree Oil as an alternative, is effective and safe for the environment.

I add 5 drops of Tea Tree Oil to each ounce of dish soap, and 20-30 drops of Tea Tree to a regular sized bucket of river water for rinse. This disinfects cutting boards, kitchen utensils, etc. Australian Tea Tree Oil is not only a "First Aid Kit in a Bottle," but an environmentally safe and effective agent for disinfectant use in the wild.

Sincerely,

Cindy Harrison,
Pagosa Springs, Colorado

Appendix

SALVE RECIPES

The first step in making a Salve is to make an Herbal Oil:

1. Powder the herbs, and place them in a 1/2 gallon glass jar. Cover herbs with oil - about two to three inches. Let sit in sun for 2 weeks, agitating every day, *OR*

2. Place powdered herbs in the top of a double boiler, and cover with oil - about 3 inches. Warm the mixture for 45 minutes, and stir as you feel necessary. For stronger infusions, let herbs steep overnight.

3. Strain the oil to remove the herbs. A piece of tightly bound cheesecloth works nicely.

4. NOTE: If using fresh herbs, follow the previous instructions, but let the herbal oil sit for an additional 2 weeks after straining. This allows the oil and water from the fresh herbs to separate. Use baster to remove water.

The basic recipe for making salve from an oil is, 1 cup oil to 1/4 cup beeswax. Once your herbal oil is ready, return it to a double boiler and add the beeswax. Heat until beeswax is melted. You can add in a variety of extras: several drops of Tea Tree Oil, with vitamin E or A, or even use a little cocoa butter in place of beeswax. Just remember the ratio of solid to liquid. Play with it. If you find the salve is too runny for you, add more beeswax. If it is hard, add a little more oil. If you plan on this salve lasting for months, Tea Tree Oil acts as a natural preservative, but you may also add a few drops of Vitamin E.

Now a word on which type of oil to use: For medicinal purposes, I like olive oil best. It usually lasts the longest. Some other alternatives are wheat germ oil or castor oil. Look for oils that are expeller pressed. This means the oils were extracted without the use of solvents. If you are making a cosmetic salve, try the lighter oils such as apricot kernel, almond, jojoba, or coconut.

(Contributed by: Leanne Deal)

MAKE SALVES WITH THESE HERBS FOR THE FOLLOWING CONDITIONS:

BRUISES

Arnica (Arnica montana) do not ingest.

Comfrey (Symphytum officinale)do not ingest

BURNS

First degree injures only the outermost layer of skin.

Second degree usually blisters and penetrates more deeply into the skin.

Third degree: seek medical assistance immediately!

Lavender: (lavandula)

Gotu Kola (Centella asiatica)

For burns use any of the herbs above, or try the following salve:

BURN SALVE: 5 oz. raw, unpasteurized honey mixed with 1 oz. Tea Tree Oil and 1 teaspoon grapefruit seed extract.

(Source: Puotinen, C.J. Natures Antiseptics: Tea Tree Oil and Grapefruit Seed Extract. New Canaan, CT; Keats Publishing, Inc., 1997).

SORES

calendula (Calendula officinalis)

comfrey (Symphytum officinale)

camomile (Matricaria recutita)

WATER MISCIBLE MIXTURES

Since Tea Tree Oil does not mix well with water, to make a formula in which Tea Tree Oil will be evenly dispersed, make a miscible formula through one of the following methods:

Add: 1 tbsp. everclear or vodka to 2 tbsp. Tea Tree Oil; shake well.

CAUTION: For External use only.

Suggested applications: Burns, cuts, athletes foot.

OR:

Add: 2 ounces vegetable glycerin to 1 ounce Tea Tree Oil. Shake well. Add 1 ounce water. Shake well again. This mixture is safe to use for topical, oral and inhalation.

Suggested applications: Douche, feet, after shave, mouthwash.

STORAGE

1. Always keep Tea Tree Oil in amber colored bottles, and store in a cool dry place.

2. Do not store in plastic bottles.

3. Cap should be on tightly to avoid oxidation and evaporation.

4. Do not store or use Tea Tree Oil near homeopathic remedies, as it may contaminate them.

5. Shelf-life is generally 2 to 3 years if properly stored.

6. Up to 20% Tea Tree Oil may be stored in Polypropylene, PVC, PET and some laminates, although stainless steel or amber is preferred.

PRECAUTIONS

1. Avoid contact with eyes.

2. Keep out of reach of children.

3. Do not take internally. This precaution does not include use with toothpaste, mouthwash (without swallowing), or douche.

4. For use in sensitive areas such as around the eyes, mouth, or genitals; dilute Tea Tree Oil with vodka or everclear, or a good grade of cold-pressed oil such as olive, apricot, almond, or avocado.

5. Dilute with cold-pressed oil before use on baby's skin.

6. Do a patch test before using Tea Tree Oil on sensitive skin. Extremely sensitive skin may need dilutions of pure oil.

Dilutions of 1:250 are bacteriostatic against pathogenic streptococci and staphylococci, typhous, pneumococcus, and gonococcus.

7. It is best to avoid alcoholic beverages (other than a glass of wine with your meal) if using essential oils.

   (Source: Better Nutrition, August 1996)

8. Pregnant women should take extra precaution, and always consult a physician.

NOTE: Use of Tea Tree Oil should not be viewed as a substitute for professional medical care. If a problem persists, consult your physician.

MATERIAL SAFETY DATA SHEET

I. Identification: Tea Tree Oil - *Melaleuca Aeternifolia*

Chemical Characteristics: Oil of Melaleuca

CAS # 68647-73-4

UN1993 Flammable Liquid nos III PG 3

II. Hazardous Ingredients

Physical Hazards: None

Health Hazards: None

(A non-hazardous material as listed under current department of labor definitions. Caution should be used by promptly disposing of oily rags, etc. to avoid the possibility of spontaneous combustion).

III. Physical Data

Appearance: Clear, colorless to pale yellow liquid, mobile at 20° C. with a myrisitic odor.

Boiling Point: N/A

Solubility in Water: Insoluble

Specific Gravity ($H_2O = 1$) : 0.90

IV. Fire and Explosion Hazard Data

Flash Point: 57-60° C (Pensky Martens closed cup IP34)

Fire Point 72° C (Cleveland open cup IP36)

Extinguishing Media: Dry chemical foam/CO_2 - *DO NOT USE WATER*

Special Fire Fighting Procedures: None Known

Unusual Fire and Explosion Hazards: None Known

V. Health Hazard Data

Toxicity; May produce toxic effect when taken internally

Health Hazards; May produce toxic side effects including seizures, coma and respiratory depression if taken internally, treatment is supportive and symptomatic, rapid absorption may be expected

VI. Reactivity Data

Stability: Stable

Incompatibility: Avoid contact with plastics, oil based paints, ink, etc. or storage in plastic.

Hazardous polymerization: Does not occur

VII. Spill or Leakage Procedure

Remove all potential sources of ignition. Contain spill with inert non-combustible absorbent material and place in approved containers.

VIII. Special Protection Information

None required

IX. Precautions for Safe Handling and Use

Store in full sealed containers in cool, dry place away from sources of ignition, heat or direct sunlight.

TEA TREE INFORMATION

Melaleuca alternifolia: common name 'tea tree." A member of the laurel tree family, unusual variety indigenous to the east coast of New South Wales, Australia. Natural stands of trees usually found in low lying, swampy areas. Trees produced from seed are now being grown on plantations in the region. Seeds are quite small, and the quality of the seed affects the output of the plantation. Seedlings take seven to ten days to germinate in the summer months; when ten to fifteen cm. tall, they are transplanted.

Essential Oil: steam-distilled essence from the root, bark, flower, and or leaf of plants. Many oils are used in healing, aromatherapy, and culinary uses.

Composition of Tea Tree Essential Oil: Naturally-occurring essential oil, colorless or pale yellow. If discolorations appear, it usually indicates an inferior distillation process. Impurities and weeds in the distillation process may also affect the color. The oil is distilled from leaves of *Melaleuca alternifolia*, consisting chiefly of terpinenes, cymenes, pinenes, terpineols, cineole, sesquiterpenes, and sequiterpen alcohols. Pleasant characteristic odor with a terebinthinate taste. If odor is strong and varies from batch to batch, it may indicate impurities at the time of distillation.

Action: Pure Tea Tree Oil conforming to Australian standard A.S.D. 175, revised 1985 (AS 2782-1985) and 1996 (ISO 4730) is a powerful broad-range antiseptic, fungicide, and bactericide. The main component is terpinen-4-ol (T-40ol). Optimal activity at 35-40% w/v. Its bacterial action is increased in the presence of blood, serum, pus, and necrotic tissue. It is able to penetrate deeply into infected tissue and pus, mix with these, and cause them to slough off while leaving a healthy surface. The oil has a very low toxicity, and is virtually a non-irritant even to sensitive tissues. Because of its lower cineole level, Tea Tree Oil is less toxic and less irritating than eucalyptus oil. Be aware that some unknown eucalyptus oils have been blended with a synthetic form of terpinen-4-ol, which alters the chemical composition.

Indications: Cuts, scratches, abrasions, burns, sunburn, prickly heat, insect bites, scalds, allergic and itching dermatoses, napkin and cosmetic rashes, senile, anal and genital pruritus, and lesions caused by herpes simplex virus including herpes labialis and herpes progenitalis. Impetigo contagiosa, furunculosis, psoriasis, and infected seborrhoeic dermatitis. Ringworm of scalp (microsporum canis), tropical ringworm (triphyton), becubitis and stasis ulcers, paronychia, oral thrush (candidiasis), tinea pedis, promidrosis, and infestation with head, body or pubic lice. As a gargle, throat spray, and nasal spray. Treatment of cutaneous staphylococcal reservoirs, boils and pimples, pyorrhea, gingivitis, halitosis, and bronchial and sinus congestion. Gynecological conditions, such as trichonomal vaginitis, moniliasis, and endocervicitis.

Precautions: Pure oil will dissolve certain plastics. Store only in glass (preferably amber) containers in a cool place. Bulk Tea Tree Oil holds up much better from damage, deterioration, and oxidization if initially stored and shipped in steel drums.

Extremely sensitive skin may need dilutions of the pure oil. Dilutions of 1:250 are still bacteriostatic against pathogenic streptococo and staphylococci, typhous, pneumococcus, and gonococcus.

Weights and Measures/Conversion Table

(Australian common usage to U.S. common usage)

1 milliliter (ml) = 0.0338/fl. ounce

10 milliliter   = 0.338/fl. ounce

1 kilogram (kg) = 2.2046 pounds

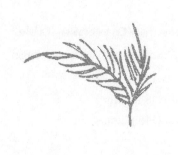

INDEX

A

Aborigines, 1
Acidophilus, 19
Acne, 9, 37
Agent Orange, 42, 63
Alcoholic beverages, 69
Alice's Wonder Spray, 43
Allergies, 8, 24, 47
Almond oil, 7, 40, 46, 60, 62, 66, 68
Aloe vera gel, 10, 16 24, 26, 33, 38
Antifungal, 1
Antiseptic, 1, 10, 37, 42, 61, 63, 72
Apricot kernel oil, 66, 68
Aquariums, 42
Arnica, 22, 62, 66
Aromatherapy, 49, 50, 57, 71
Arthrits, 21, 29
Aspirin, 21
Athletes foot, 27, 67
Avocado oil, 62, 68

B

Baby care, 1, 53
Baking soda, 15, 50, 60, 61
Bandage, 27, 28, 30, 59, 61, 62
Bath oil(s), 2, 49
Bath salts, 50
Bath, 3, 61 17, 22, 25, 33, 38, 50, 55, 56
Beauty care, 37
Bedsores, 46
Beeswax, 65, 66
Bladder infection, 31
Bleach, 44, 46
Blisters, 11, 22, 24, 27, 55, 59, 61, 66
Body lotion, 28, 38, 40
Body smoother, 38
Borax, 43, 45, 46, 50
Bottles, 50
Breasts, 34, 57
Bronchial congestion, 17, 73
Bronchitis, 17
Bruises, 22, 66

Brushing, Dry, 38
Burdock, 14

C

Calamine lotion, 53, 55, 60
Calendula salve, 54, 55
Calendula, 9, 24, 54, 67
Camomile, 67
Camping, 10, 59, 60, 63
Candida albicans, 19, 34
Canker sores, 10
Carbolic acid, 42
Carcinogenic, 5, 44
Carrot seed oil, 23, 50
Castor oil, 66
Chamomile oil, 9, 47
Chapped lips, 10
Cheesecloth, 65
Chemicals, 24, 44
Chest, 17
Chicken pox, 53
Child care, 53
Chlorinated phosphates, 44
Chlorine, 64
Citronella, 60

Clay, 22, 37, 38, 39, 60
Cocoa butter, 65
Coconut oil, 66
Cold sores, 11
Colds, 3, 54
Comfrey, 22, 32, 66, 67
Complex phosphates, 44
Compress, 21, 22, 32, 49, 62
Constipation, 32
Corns and calluses, 28
Cortisone, 21
Cosmetic salve, 66
Cosmetics, 49
Cough, 17, 18, 56
Cradle cap, 54
Cuticles, 40
Cuts, 1, 24, 67, 72
Cutting boards, 64
Cystitis, 31

D

Dandruff, 5, 6
Deodorant, 1, 37
Deodorizer, 50, 57
Dermatitis, 23, 24, 54, 72

Diaper cleanser, 54

Diaper rash, 54

Diarrhea, 58

Disinfectant, 42, 64

Disinfectant, hand, 46

Disinfectant, room, 57

Douche, 34, 67

Dr. Bronner's, 63

Dry skin, 29, 39, 50

E

Ear infection, 3, 6, 55

Earache, 6, 55

Eczema, 23, 24

EDTA, 44

Emphysema, 17

Environment, 41, 42, 44, 64

F

Face, 8, 9, 11, 38, 39, 54, 55

Facial mask, 39, 49

Fire ant bites, 59

Flu, 47

Foot balm, 1

Fungus, 19, 27, 37, 40, 45

G

Gangrene, diabetic, 28, 29

Genitals, 68

Geriatric, 28

Gingivitis, 14, 73

Glycerin, 7, 8, 10, 67

Glycol, 44

Gold shots, 21

Gonococcus, 69, 73

Gotu Kola, 67

Gout, 29

Grapeseed oil, 17, 18, 22, 23, 24, 25, 28, 29, 33, 39, 60

Green clay, 60

Gums, receeding/bleeding, 13, 14

Gums, sore, bad breath, 15

H

Hair and Follicles, cleansing, 5

Hair conditioner, 50

Hair, dry or oily, 6

Hair, ingrown, 10, 35

Hair rinse, 51

Head, 2, 5, 6, 18, 54, 73

Head cold, 7

Head lice, 7

Headache, 8, 44, 47

Heat rash, 55

Hemorrhoids, 32

Herpes, 11, 33, 53, 72

Hives, 24

Home care, 2, 41, 46

Homeopathic remedies, 68

Horsetail, 14

Hospital, 28, 35, 46, 58

Humidifier, 18, 47, 50, 57

Hydrogen peroxide, 42, 45, 46

I

ICE, 62

Immune system, 30, 57

Impetigo, 55, 72

Ingrown hairs, 10, 35

Insect bites, 55, 60, 61, 72

Insect repellent, 2, 60

Insects, 45, 60

Iodine, 40

J

Jock itch, 33

Jojoba oil, 21, 22, 23, 25, 26, 49, 50, 51, 66

K

Kitchen utensils, 42, 64

L

Lavender oil, 24, 39, 47, 53, 61, 66

Leeches, 60, 61

Leg toner, 35

Leg ulcers, 29

Legs and feet, 27

Lemon, 47

Lice, 7, 72

Lungs, 17

Lyme's disease, 62

M

Massage, 1, 3, 6, 8, 15, 17, 22, 23, 24, 25, 28, 29 33, 37, 38, 40, 46, 47, 49, 51, 57, 61

Measles, 56

Memory, 47

Microorganisms, 14, 41

Mineral oil, 9, 38

Molds, 45

Mood, 47

Morpholine, 44

Mouthwash, 2, 14, 15, 16, 18, 19, 67, 68

Muscle aches, 24, 50

Myrrh, 14, 30

N

Nail Infections, 40

Nail Soak, 40

Nail Stains, 40

Nasal Ulcer, 8

Neem, 14

Neroli oil, 37, 39

Nicotinia glutinosa, 45

Nursing, home care, 46

O

Oatmeal, 53

Oatmeal soap, 61

Olive oil, 6, 7, 27, 28, 40, 46, 54, 55, 66, 68

On the Road, 41

Outdoors, 59, 60

Osteo Arthrits, 21

Ovarian Cysts, 33

Oxidation, 68

P

PABA, 62

Papillomavirus, 30

Patch test, 68

Pathogenic streptococci, 69, 73

Peppermint oil, 60

Perfume body mist, 51

Perfumes, 49, 50

Perionychia, 40

Peroxide, 16

Personal hygiene, 31, 63

PET, 68

Petroleum based, 38, 44, 55

Plantar Warts, 30

Plants, 18, 24, 41, 45, 71

Plaque, 13, 14, 15

Plastics, 50, 70, 73

Pneumococcus, 69, 73

Poison ivy/oak/sumac, 61

Polypropylene, 68

Poultice, 22

Precautions, 68, 71, 73

Pregnant, 32, 69

Propyl alcohol, 5

Psoriasis, 25, 72

PVC, 68

R

Radon gas, 41

Rash, skin, 55

Rheumatoid Arthrits, 21

Ringworm of Scalp, 25, 72

Ringworm of Skin, 26

Ringworm, 25, 72

Room freshener, 47

Rosemary oil, 37, 47, 50

S

Salt, sea, 14, 15, 18, 25, 50, 56, 57

Salve, 11, 22, 23, 24, 27, 28, 32, 54, 55, 59, 60, 65, 66, 67

Sandalwood oil, 50

Sandfleas, 61

Saunas, 49

Shaving, 10

Sinusitis, 8

Skin, dry, 29, 39, 50

Slippery elm, 18, 19

Soap, 2, 9, 23, 24, 27, 28, 33, 37, 42, 43, 46, 61, 63, 64

Sodium bromide, 44

Sodium laurel sulphate, 5

Splinters, 61

Sprains, 61

Stainless steel, 68

Staph aureus, 46

Staphylococcus bacteria, 55

Staphylococci, 11, 69, 73

Steam inhaler, 7, 8, 56

Stinger, 60

Stings, 60, 61

Storage, 68, 70

Streptococcoal bacteria, 57, 69

Stye, 11

Sunburn, 62, 63, 72

Sunscreen, 2, 37

Suppositories, 1, 33

T

Tarter, 14

Teeth, 12, 14, 15, 16

Thinning hair, 5

Throat and chest, 17

Throat lozenges, 18, 19

Throat, sore, 3, 18, 56, 57

Throat, strep, 18

Thrush, 19, 34, 72

Thyme oil, 37

Tick fever, 62

Ticks, 3, 62

Tiger Balm, 24, 25

Tobacco virus, 45

Tonsillitis, 57

Toothache, 16

Toothbrush care, 14, 15, 16

Toothpaste, 2, 14, 15, 68

Toxicity, 58, 70, 72

Triclosan, 42

Tumor, Epithelical, 30

Tweezers, 28, 61, 62, 63

Typhous, 69, 73

U

Urethra, 21, 31

V

Vaginitis, 34, 73

Vaporizer, 7, 8, 18, 19, 47, 50, 51, 53, 54, 56, 57

Vaseline, 38, 55

Vegetable glycerin, 67

Vegetable oil, 5

Veterinarian, 2

Vetivert oil, 50

Vinegar, 43

Virus, 41, 45, 53, 56, 57, 72

Vitamin E, 33, 57, 62, 65, 66

Vodka, 7, 8, 33, 45, 67, 68

W

Warts, 3, 26, 30

Washing machine, 8, 46

Water miscible, 54, 67

Water, Distilled, 31, 34, 42, 43, 47

Waxing, 10, 35

Wheat germ oil, 40, 66

Witch hazel, 9, 24, 32, 35, 55, 56

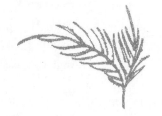

ABOUT THE AUTHOR

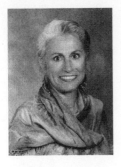

Cynthia Olsen is the author of several books, and a successful publisher, researcher and speaker on complementary health, healing and spiritual awareness. In addition to her role as mother and grandmother, she is a successful entrepreneur and business-person, and a lifelong supporter and exponent of holistic living. Her managerial experience in the health food industry in the 1980s led her to form an import company, becoming a leading figure in the introduction of Australian Tea Tree Oil to the American health scene.

In 1990, Ms. Olsen founded Kali Press, a publishing house committed to works addressing the full spectrum of life awareness, with concentration on natural healing modalities. Her book *Essiac: A Native Herbal Cancer Remedy*, won the Small Press Book Award in 1997. The book has now gone into second edition.

Ms. Olsen's books have been translated into other languages. She has appeared on television, radio, and has addressed various conventions and meetings on health and natural living.

From her Colorado home, she continues to actively pursue her varied interests in nature and the spirit of joyful living.

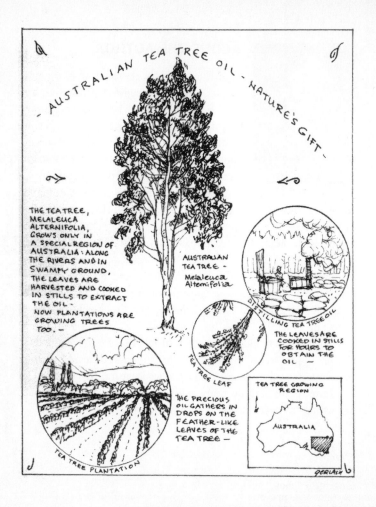

- AUSTRALIAN TEA TREE OIL - NATURE'S GIFT -

THE TEA TREE, MELALEUCA ALTERNIFOLIA, GROWS ONLY IN A SPECIAL REGION OF AUSTRALIA: ALONG THE RIVERS AND IN SWAMPY GROUND. THE LEAVES ARE HARVESTED AND COOKED IN STILLS TO EXTRACT THE OIL - NOW PLANTATIONS ARE GROWING TREES TOO. -

AUSTRALIAN TEA TREE - Melaleuca Alternifolia

DISTILLING TEA TREE OIL

THE LEAVES ARE COOKED IN STILLS FOR HOURS TO OBTAIN THE OIL -

TEA TREE LEAF

THE PRECIOUS OIL GATHERS IN DROPS ON THE FEATHER-LIKE LEAVES OF THE TEA TREE -

TEA TREE GROWING REGION

AUSTRALIA

TEA TREE PLANTATION

GERLACH

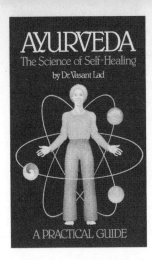

AYURVEDA: THE SCIENCE OF SELF-HEALING
Dr. Vasant Lad
175 pp pb $10.95
ISBN 0-914955-00-4

For the first time a book is available which clearly explains the principles and practical applications of Ayurveda, the oldest healing system in the world. This beautifully illustrated text thoroughly explains history & philosophy, basic principles, diagnostic techniques, treatment, diet, medicinal usage of kitchen herbs & spices, first aid, food aid, food antidotes and much more.

More than 50 concise charts, diagrams and tables are included, as well as a glossary and index in order to further clarify the text.

YOGA FOR YOUR TYPE
Dr. David Frawley &
Sandra Summerfield Kozak, M.S.
296 pp os $29.95
ISBN 0-910261-30-X

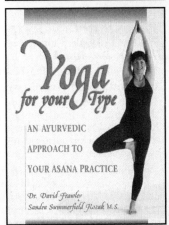

This is the first book that details how to choose Yoga asanas (Yoga poses) most appropriate for your unique body type according to the five thousand year old system of Ayurvedic medicine. These two systems of healing and energy management have long been regarded as effective methods of relieving stress, creating personal balance, eliminating ailments, and relieving chronic pain. *Yoga for Your Type* presents a fundamental understanding of both Yoga and Ayurveda and provides the information needed for you to balance your energy and feel healthy.

"By reading this book, you will be able to personalize your yoga program and gain maximum benefit in integrating body, mind and spirit as one experience of consciousness."
—Deepak Chopra, M.D., Author of *Grow Younger Live Longer*

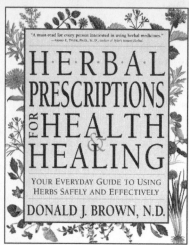

HERBAL PRESCRIPTIONS FOR HEALTH & HEALING
Donald J. Brown, N.D.

464 pp os $24.95

ISBN 0-940985-58-6

UPC 0 79565 02091 4

For centuries, herbal medicine has offered safe, inexpensive, and effective ways to treat a wide variety of health conditions. *Herbal Prescriptions for Health and Healing* is an indispensable guide that will introduce you to 20 of the most frequently used herbs. The book also provides extensive information on treating all the primary systems of the body with herbal medicine. Whether you're a novice or an experienced herb user, you'll find many helpful tips for a wide variety of ailments, including: arthritis, colds and flus, diabetes, memory loss, prostate enlargement and many more!

THE SPIRIT OF REIKI
Walter Lübeck, Frank Arjava Petter, William Lee Rand

312 pp pb $19.95   ISBN 0-914955-67-5

150 photos and b/w illustrations

Written by three world-renowned Reiki masters, this book is a first. Never before have three Reiki masters from different lineages and with extensive backgrounds come together to share their experience.

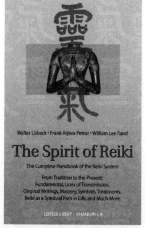

The Spirit of Reiki contains a wealth of information on Reiki never before brought together in one place. The broad spectrum of topics range from the search for a scientific explanation of Reiki energy to Reiki as a spiritual path. It includes the latest understanding of Dr. Usui's original healing methods, how Reiki is currently practiced in Japan, an analysis of the Western evolution of Reiki, and a discussion about the direction Reiki is likely to take in the future.